OXYNOW

LUXURY
WE CANNOT
AFFORD

BREATH AWARENESS
&
OXYGEN

Breath and oxygen are a sure thing in our life, why we would even bother to write this book talking about these 2 things that have been in our life since the start of our lives till the end of it?

Because the breath and oxygen are such a sure thing, we don't give it any attention. Yet every day we breathe less and less oxygen than it was usual ever before. It's because of the shallow breathing and air pollution. The less oxygen we get with each inhalation we do, the more this can affect us in a matter of 5,10, or 15 in our health. It might be the death of a thousand cuts.

On the other hand, mindful conscious breathing can improve significantly our everyday life as well as our mental and physical health.

Content

Introduction

Breath is life

This book is about breath and how a simple thing like breath awareness and oxygen is able to help us to connect with ourselves and the World around us. You are already here, you read these words, and you breathe the oxygen around you, how else you would live if you couldn't breathe? That's the thing, we breathe, or more likely to say, our body and subconscious mind are breathing automatically based on evolution and that is what we thought over the years of our life. Because breathing is such a simple thing, our mind tends to overlook it and thus it thinks that such a thing as a breath doesn't need any more attention because it's already going fully automatic and without problem.

First of all, let's introduce oxygen a little bit. Oxygen is a chemical element with an atomic number of 8 (it has eight protons in its nucleus). Oxygen forms a molecule (O2) of two atoms which is a colorless gas at normal temperatures and pressures. If you think about it this way even though it's the true core of it, it's pretty boring and complicated to say it out loud this way. Let's try it differently.

Without food, we can survive several weeks, without water for several days, and without oxygen for several minutes. Yes, this makes it sounds better and sprinkles a lil bit of drama over this cake. It's like that, without oxygen we cannot survive more than maybe 1,2 or 3 minutes, after this period we lose our consciousness and if we don't get the oxygen supply 5-10 minutes after that, we are done living in this beautiful place we call Earth. This makes oxygen the real "Food of Life", the biggest necessity for us to thrive.

Oxygen fuels our cells and helps provide the basic building block our bodies need to survive. Our cells combine oxygen with nitrogen and hydrogen to produce various proteins that build new cells. Oxygen is also necessary for constructing replacement cells for our bodies. Every day, about seven hundred billion cells in our body wear out and must be replaced. Without oxygen, our body cannot build these new cells.

Oxygen plays a particularly important part of our immune system. It is used to help kill bacteria and it fuels the cells that make up our body's defenses against viruses and other invaders.

So Oxygen helps organisms grow, reproduce and turn food into energy. Humans get the oxygen they need by breathing through our nose and mouth into the lungs. Oxygen gives our cells the ability to break down food in order to get the energy we need to survive.

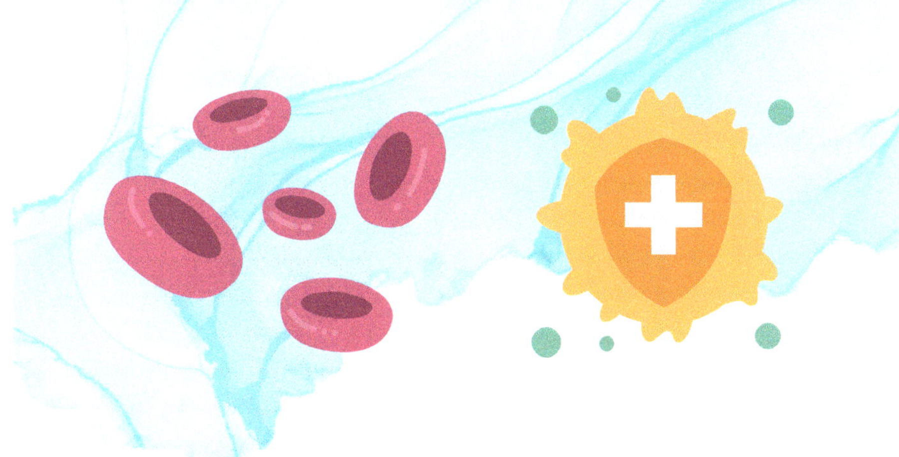

5 ways our body is able to absorb oxygen into the body.

Each of them does a different function and works differently.

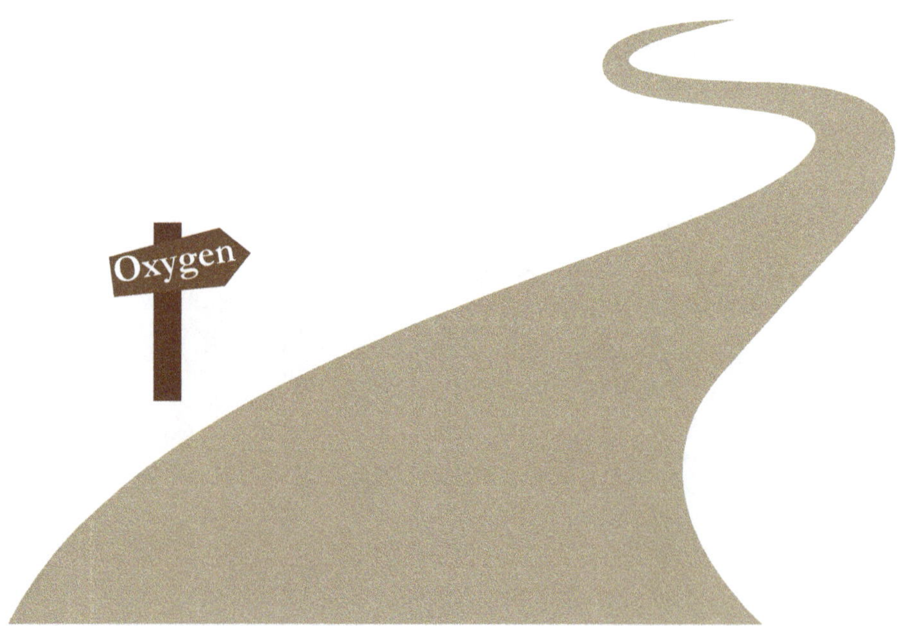

The human eye

You are not crazy, you see it correctly. Without this precious gas, the human eye will work. The eye receives oxygen in a manner that is unique from the rest of the body. The cornea is built in such a way to diffuse oxygen directly into the body from the air.

Because there is no presence of blood vessels in the eyes, they need to get oxygen from the other source. They get it directly from the atmosphere. The eye can consume oxygen only at a certain rate. It's the inner part of the eye (The Endothelium), that needs oxygen. The endothelium is a monolayer of cells on the posterior corneal surface that transports water from the stroma into the anterior chamber. It is the main mechanism of repair after cell loss.

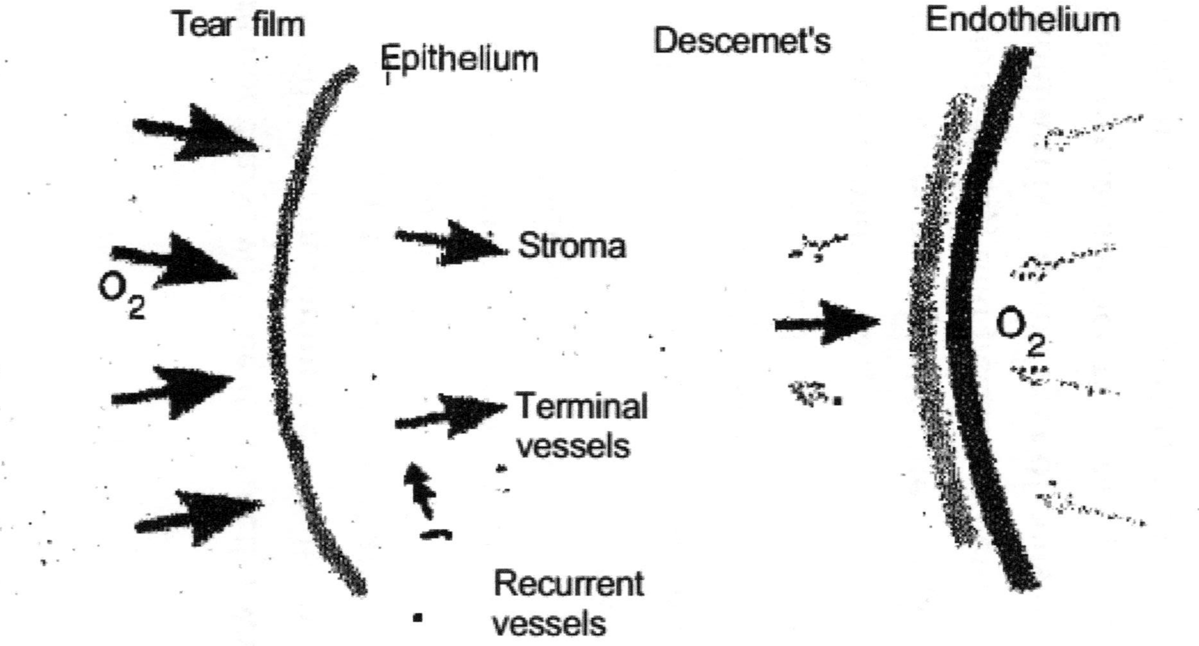

ATMOSPHERE
AQUEOUS HUMOR
Tear film
Epithelium
Descemet's
Endothelium
Stroma
Terminal vessels
Recurrent vessels
O2
O2

Stomach and digestive system

a.k.a.

by oxygenated water

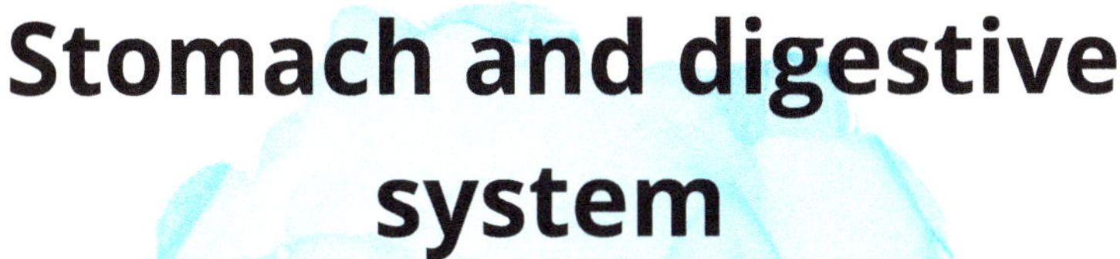

Oxygenated water, or "hydrogenated water," has extra oxygen added to water during the bottling process. It has several benefits beyond the usual benefit of drinking water. Oxygenated water is made by increasing the atmospheric pressure around the water so that the level of dissolved water increases. Oxygenated water may help to sober you up after drinking a large amount of alcohol, a small study found that drinking oxygenated water could be beneficial in speeding up alcohol metabolism. It is beneficial to consume during and after exercise since the extra oxygen in the body helps to get rid of lactic acid more effectively. This oxygen absorption is through the stomach and digestive system.

Skin

Skin cells absorb oxygen from and release carbon dioxide into the surrounding air. The amount of oxygen that diffuses through the skin is negligible, a tiny percentage of what we absorb through the lungs. Still, it's enough to supply a significant amount of the oxygen needs of your skin's surface layer, the epidermis. The epidermis is like a thin coat of paint on the much thicker, deeper layer of the skin called the dermis. The dermis has a blood supply, but the epidermis doesn't. You can influence the blood supply to your skin indirectly. When you practice asana and your muscles heat up, more blood flows to the skin to dissipate the heat.

The skin is the only organ besides the lungs that is directly exposed to atmospheric oxygen. Oxygen is consumed in all layers of the epidermis and dermis.

Then there is another very well-known way to get oxygen into our body, some call it a myth, some call it an illusion, and some call it a necessity. There have been countless books written about it and businesses built around it. One that can be translated into various languages as a life. It's a way to cure a lot of physical and mental issues, it's a way to feel this moment and the real flow of time and life. You guessed it.

I am talking about THE BREATH.

The Breath

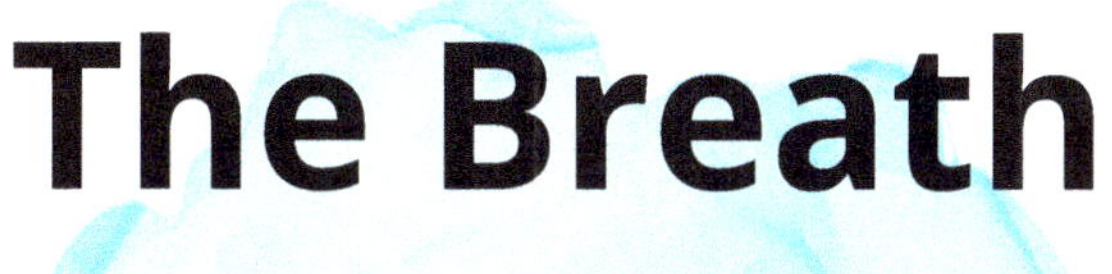

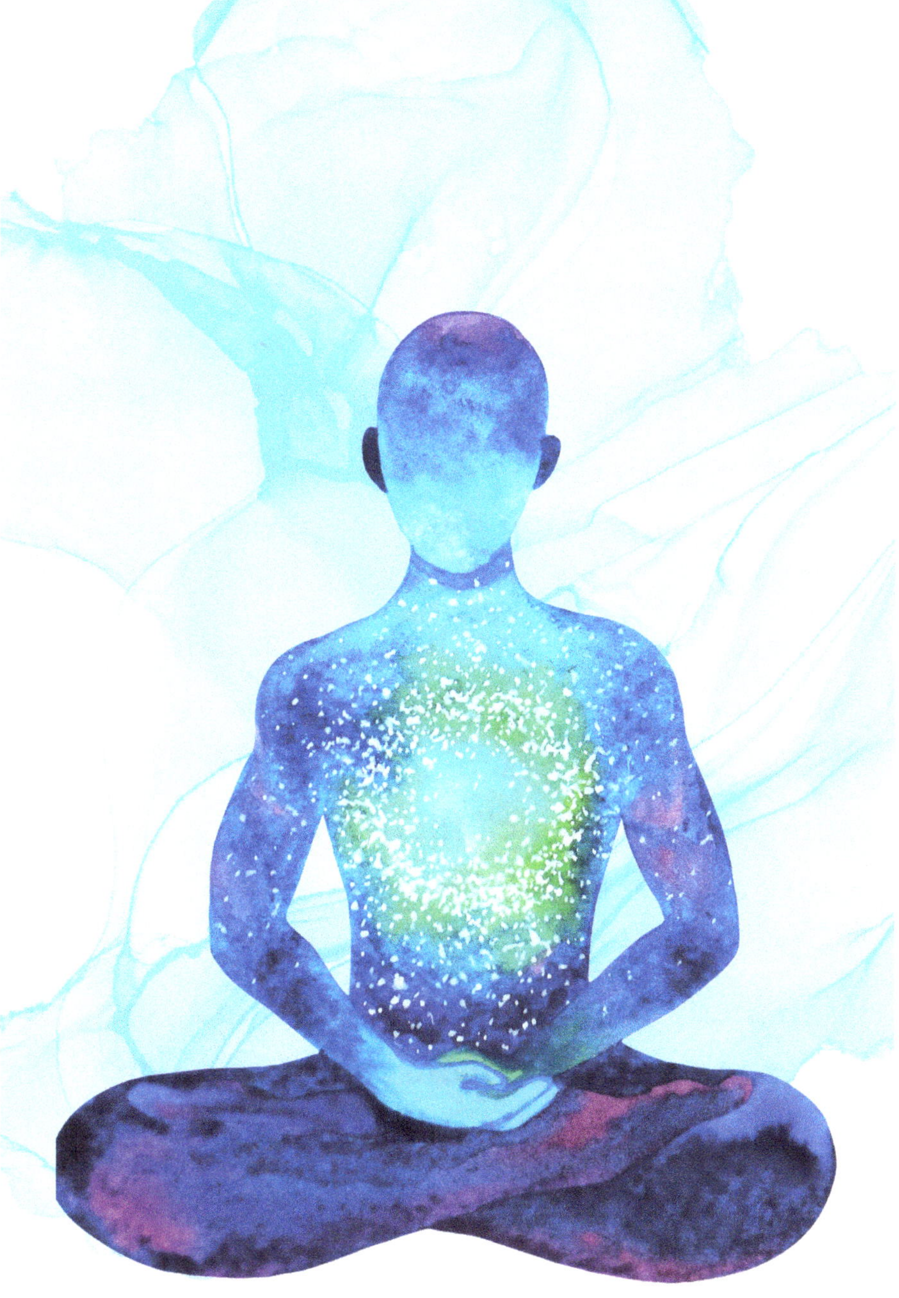

What is breath?

The most basic definition is a welcome of a refreshing change. Breath secures the most important body exchange we need. Support our body with fresh new oxygen and release the dangerous carbon dioxide from our body.

Breath is the force that sustains life and conscious breath is the force that sustains awareness. In the practices of yoga, the breath is fundamental, as well for life, because it's the main gateway for the oxygen to enter our body.

Regulated breath opens the body and channels vital energy or prana. Conscious breath provides focus and enables the mind to reach its meditative state. The control of breath is also known as pranayama in Sanskrit.

The normal respiratory rate for an adult at rest is 12 to 18 breaths per minute. The speed, pattern, and depth of your breath indicate how well your body is working to deliver oxygen to all your vital organs and tissues. Your respiratory rate can be affected by many different factors such as alcohol consumption, sleep apnea, infections, or heart conditions.

What is a respiratory rate measure?

It's a metabolic process of oxygen intake and carbon dioxide release. It's controlled by a body system called the respiratory drive.

- **Neural central control: The NCC system sets the ventilation rate and air intake volume. This affects exhalation, inhalation, and breathing pattern.**

- **Sensory input system: The sensory system sends information back to the central nervous system to indicate how much volume and at what rate to breathe. It also recognizes chemical changes such as irritants.**

- **Muscular system: The muscular system moves the lungs in accordance with signals from the other systems. It controls the mechanic of breathing.**

These systems work together to create a process that exchanges oxygen and carbon dioxide. When we breathe out, we release low oxygen and high carbon dioxide. When we breathe in, we take in high oxygen and low carbon dioxide. The exchange of these elements is important for metabolic processes to continue at the cellular level.

Carbon dioxide is an odorless, colorless gas. It is a waste product that your body makes when it uses food for energy. Your blood carries carbon dioxide to your lungs. When you exhale, you breathe out carbon dioxide.CO2 plays various roles in the human body including regulation of blood pH, respiratory drive, and affinity of hemoglobin for oxygen (O2).

We breathe in 2 particular ways

Mouth breathing vs Nose breathing

Breathing is breathing, the important thing is that we can get so much highlighted oxygen to our body so we don't die and can live up to the other day. Is it something that you've heard or that the voice whispers back in your head?

It's true, you are going live no matter what style of breathing you're going to choose. Just to be honest, one way is more pleasant than the other. One of them has the potential to make a positive trace in our life, the other one not so much. One has the potential to improve the quality of each day, without any effort, the other one does the opposite, without any effort.

One of them has the potential to save your marriage, and the other one will contribute to the separation. One of them has the potential to heal your mental health problems, the other one is making them more powerful. The positive side brings out only the nose breathing. The negative is caused by mouth breathing.

Am I pulling up your leg? Creating this crap as I move on with this text? Is this garbage from the depth of a trash can of another company selling you its perspective and ideology?

None of those, even though we sold you this e-book. What you will take out of it is only up to you. That, what you bought is a material that has the great potential to improve the quality of your life, save the precious commodity we have in this life which is time and protect your health.

Back to the mouth breathing...

Why it should be a thing for you to be concerned about?

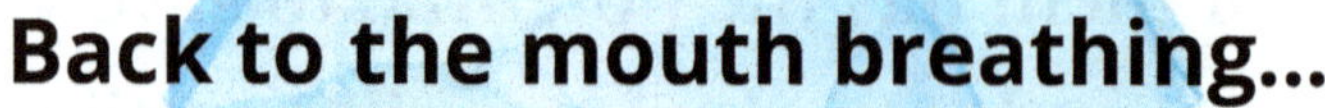

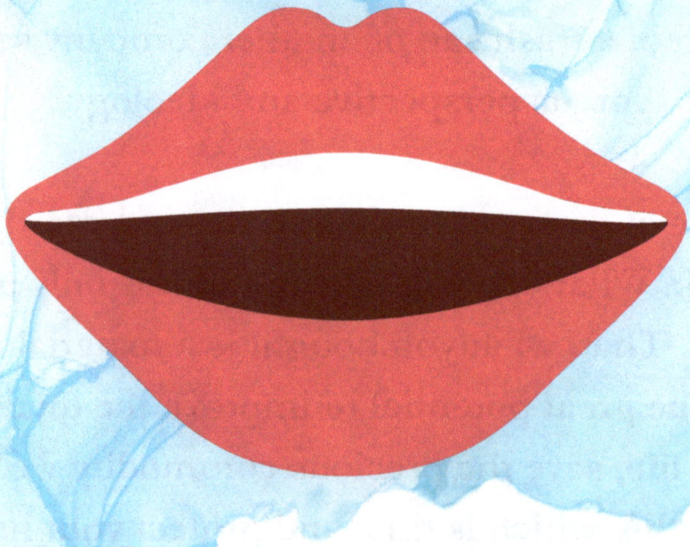

Mouth breathing has been shown to increase the propensity for upper airway collapse. The most likely explanation is that jaw opening is associated with a posterior movement of the angle of the jaw, which compromises the oropharynx airway diameter. The oropharynx is the middle part of your throat (pharynx) just beyond your mouth. it also includes the tonsils, the base of your tongue, the dyes and walls of your throat, and the back part of the roof of your mouth.

Breathing through the mouth all the time, especially when you are sleeping can lead to problems. In children, mouth breathing causes crooked teeth, facial deformities, or poor growth. In adults, chronic mouth breathing can cause bad breath and gum disease. It can also worsen symptoms of other illnesses.

How do I know if I am breathing through my mouth?

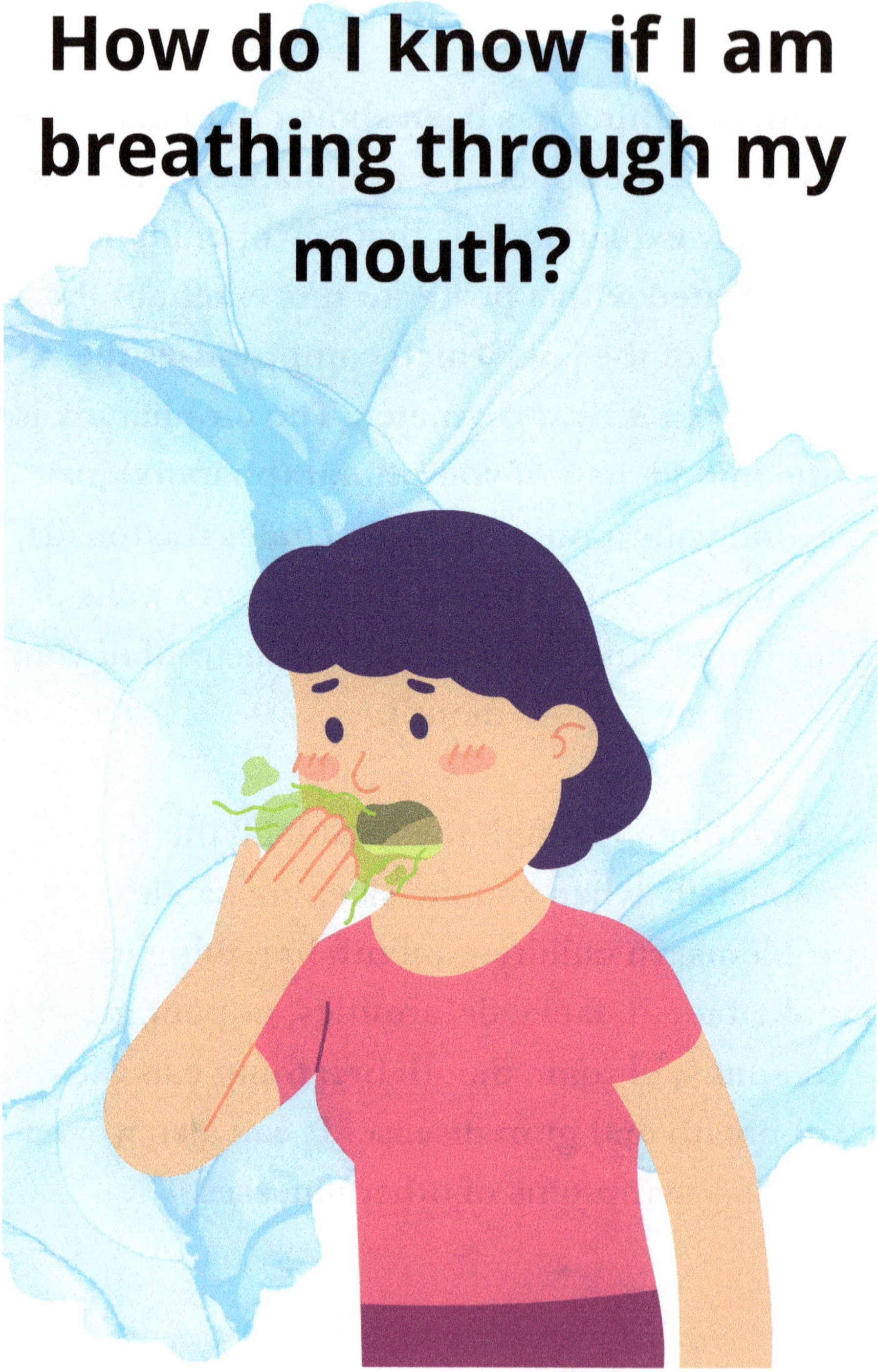

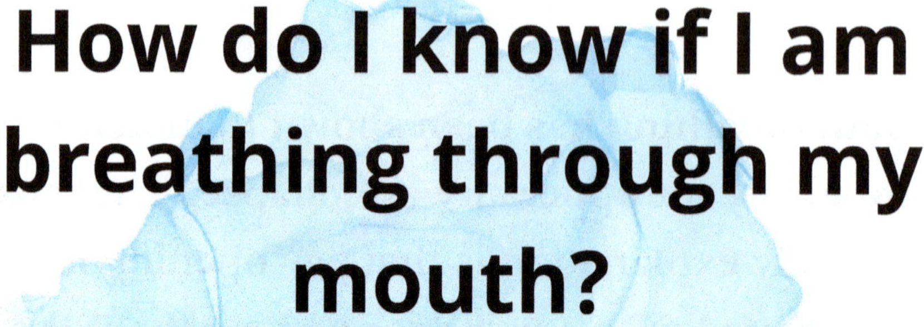

30 to 50% of adults breathe through their mouth, especially earlier in the day.

Many people don't realize they are breathing by their mouth instead of their nose, especially if it happens when they are sleeping. There is a range of factors that can cause mouth breathing. The cause might be obstructed partially or completely blocked nasal airway. Essentially, something stands in the way of smooth airflow into the nasal passage. This pattern activates the sympathetic nervous system leading to shallow, rapid, and abnormal breathing. That's one of the reasons that creates anxiety, depression, and stress in our bodies.

Chronic mouth breathing is associated with several health complications and while an individual will not necessarily experience all of the symptoms or complications, they may have one or several of them.

These symptoms are usually the key, which unlocks the knowledge about this behavior.

Snoring
A dry mouth
Bad breath
A hoarse voice
Brain fog
Waking up tired and irritable
Chronic fatigue
Sleep disorders like insomnia
Dark circles under the eyes
A slightly open mouther appearance
Being a "noisy" eater

For children it might be:

Irritability
problems concentrating at school
increasing crying episodes at night
dry, cracked lips
a strong mouth odor

In children, the harmful effects of mouth breathing are far greater, since it is during these formative years that breathing mode helps to shape the orofacial structures and airways. Children whose mouth breathing is left untreated for extended periods of time can set the stage for lifelong respiratory problems. As a result, malocclusions such as a skeletal Class II or Class III, along with a long lower face height, also characterized as "long face syndrome", and high palatal vaults may also be noted.

Before and after surgery for long face syndrome

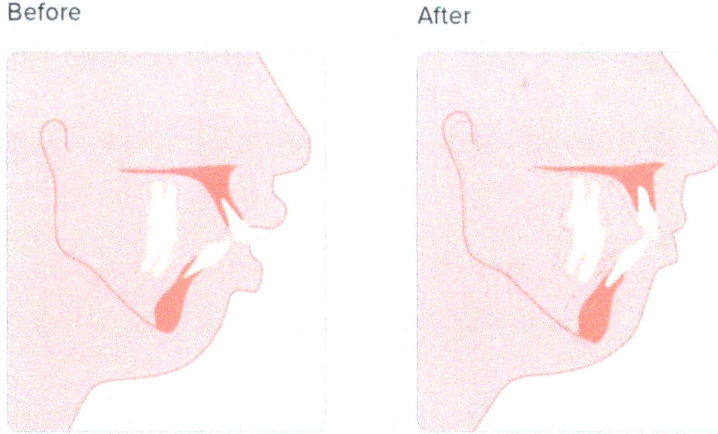

International Journal of Pediatrics investigating the long-term changes to facial structure caused by chronic mouth breathing noted that this seemingly "benign" habit has in fact immediate and latent cascading effects on multiple physiological and behavioral functions. Mouth breathing can have a tremendous impact on the mental and physical health of children: As it can be associated with the restriction of the lower airways, poor quality of sleep, reduced cognitive functioning, and a lower quality of life

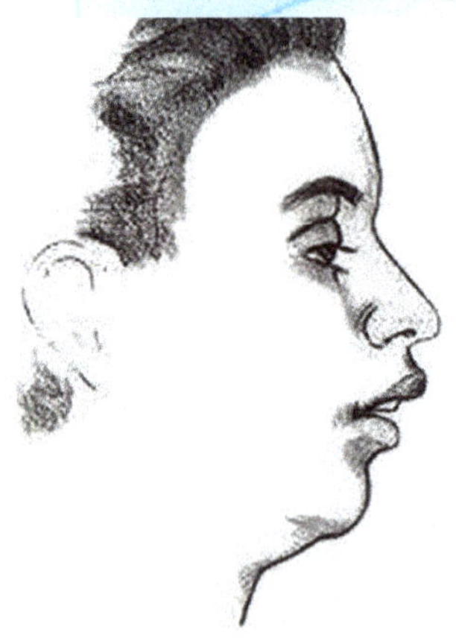

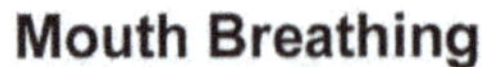

Mouth Breathing

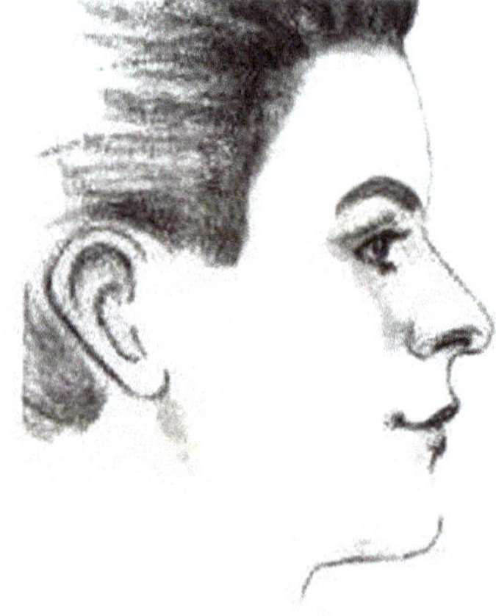

Nose Breathing

How can mouth breathing affect you in the long term?

Mouth breathing directly affects behavioral performance and dental health. Previous studies have observed that oral breathing can increase the likelihood of brain functional problems due to lower oxygen saturation in the human brain. Recent studies have demonstrated an association between mouth breathing and cognitive deficits. Significant decreases in memory and learning ability during oral breathing, and changes in the central nervous system in animal research. In addition, there was a decline in working memory performance for specific cognitive tasks in children with oral breathing and for olfactory memory tasks caused by oral breathing in healthy adults. Furthermore, changes in brain function, including oxygen load and brain activity during oral breathing, have been demonstrated in a variety of ways.

Previous studies have shown that oral breathing could change the default mode network and create more widespread brain functional connectivity in oral breathing conditions than in nasal breathing conditions during the resting state.

It might be the gateway to the development of a sleep-breathing disorder, even in your children. A sleep breathing disorder, such as obstructive sleep apnea, means frequent disruptions of the sleep cycle and low oxygen levels.

A mouth breather carries the tongue in a low downward position, creating an airspace that allows the person to breathe more freely, as a result, it can lead to abnormal tongue activity. This abnormal activity can exert an excessive force upon the dentition during swallowing, contributing to malocclusions in children and leading to periodontal disease and atypical myofascial pain in adulthood.

Low tongue resting posture can contribute to various morphological changes to the orofacial structures. And consequently, Orofacial Myofunctional Disorders (OMDs) may develop as well, they can, directly and indirectly, affect chewing, swallowing, speech, occlusion, temporomandibular joint movement, oral hygiene, stability of orthodontic treatment, facial aesthetics, facia skeletal growth.

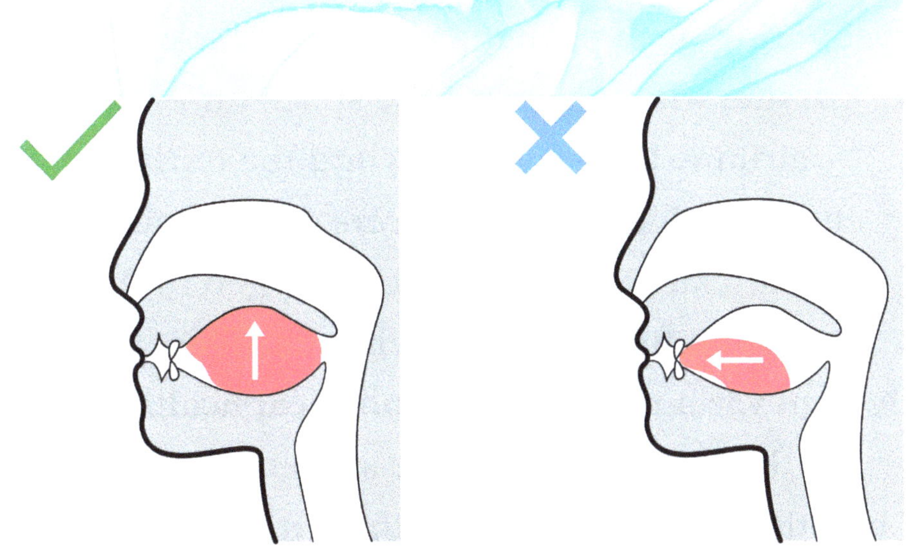

Snoring and sleep apnea

Snoring is the sound that results from air passing through your airway when it is partially blocked. Tissues at the top of your airway touch each other and vibrate, which causes snoring. Snoring knows or experiences almost everyone is this Earth. This sound can be unbearable and might disrupt the sleep of everyone in the household.

It's very common for married couples to sleep separately due to loud and unpleasant snoring. Snoring occurs when the airways have loose tissue, which narrows the space for proper airflow. It goes way beyond the terrible chainsaw-like sound. Snorers actually receive significantly less amount of oxygen in their bodies compared to non snorers. This might lead to various mental and physical health issues in the long term because snorers primarily breathe through their mouths during the night.

Does the thought of snoring gives you goosebumps and it digs out all of the moments when you have been furious about it when you couldn't get a quality sleep?

Snoring is often associated with a sleep disorder called obstructive sleep apnea. Not all snorers have OSA, but if snoring is accompanied by any following symptoms, it may be an indication to see a doctor for further observation:

- Witnessed breathing pauses during sleep
- Excessive daytime sleepiness
- Difficulty concentrating
- Morning headaches
- Sore throat upon awakening
- Restless sleep
- Gasping or choking at night
- High blood pressure
- Chest pain at night
- Your snoring is so loud it's disrupting your partner's sleep

It's often characterized by a loud snoring followed by a period of silence when breathing stops or nearly stops. Eventually, this reduction or pause in breathing may signal you to wake up, and you may awaken with a loud snort or gasping sound. You may sleep lightly due to disrupted sleep. This pattern of breathing pauses may be repeated many times during the night.

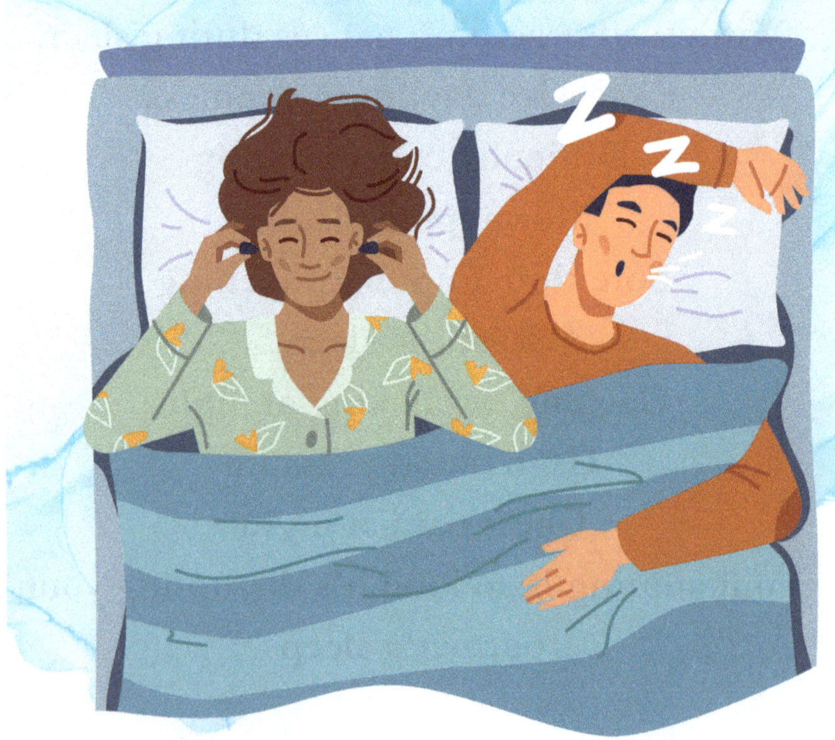

How to get rid of snoring?

If you or your partner snore regularly, you might wonder how to stop snoring. You are definitely not alone in this. From the overall population, 44% of men snore and 28% of women snore. This number is growing with each year. Different people snore for different reasons.

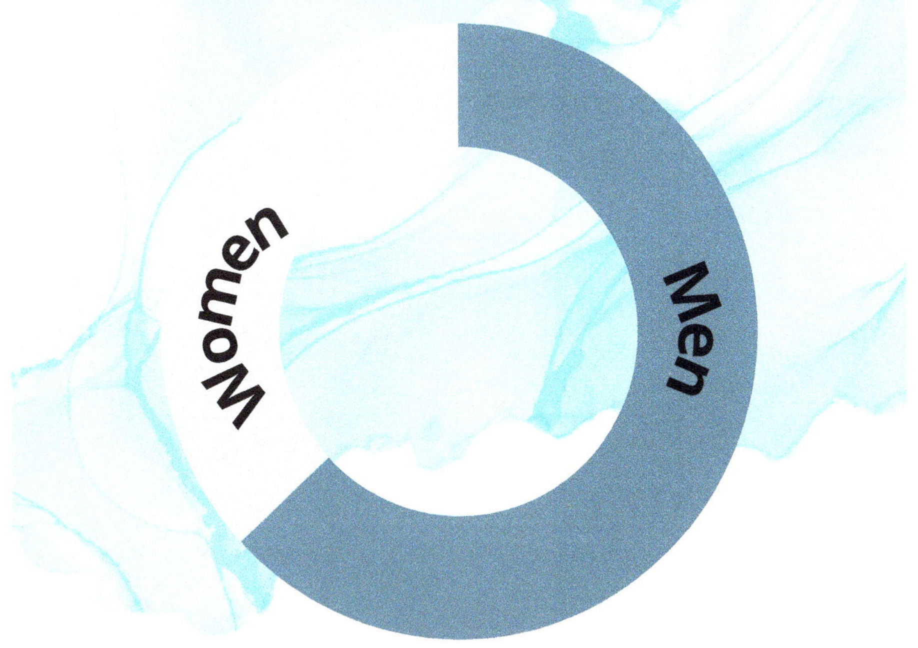

Change your sleeping position

Your snoring might depend on what position you sleep in. People are more likely to snore when sleeping on their backs, also called the supine position. People snore less, when they sleep on their sides, which is called a lateral position. The tendency to snore could be more due to head position than body position.

Reduce body weight

Experts recommend weight loss as one of the first and most important treatments to try for snoring. Of course, this recommendation only applies to people who are overweight and obese. 74% of Americans are overweight or obese, people with obesity are more likely to snore and to develop obstructive sleep apnea. Research has found that weight loss in people with a high body mass index reduces both, snoring and obstructive sleep apnea symptoms. So if you decide to approach weight loss, do it in a healthy way. Crash diets rarely work in a long term.

Try mouth exercises

In addition to exercising generally, consider mouth exercises to stop snoring. Clinically, these exercises are known as oropharyngeal exercises, have been found to effectively reduce snoring.
Mouth exercises involve repeatedly moving your tongue and party of your mouth in ways that strengthen muscles in the tongue, soft palate, and throat. 3 months of study exercises could lead to a 59% reduction in snoring.

Consider surgical treatments

Snoring sometimes results from physical issues that medical professionals can resolve through surgery. Although surgery should be viewed as a last resort, there are few surgeries that are known to reduce snoring. But this option is quite drastic and often very expensive.

Quit smoking

Smoking cigarettes is associated with increased snoring. So quitting smoking can help with your snoring problem. Additionally, children of parents who smoke tend to snore more.
Avoid alcohol before bed

Not only does alcohol increase snoring, but drinking before bed can even induce obstructive sleep apnea in people who don't have the disorder. Alcohol's effect on snoring and sleep is dose-related, so if you tend to drink multiple drinks, start by cutting back.

Consider using Nasal strips

Using nasal strips is a convenient and easy way how to minimalize snoring to a minimum without spending thousands of dollars on surgeries and going under the procedures. Nasal strips open up the nasal wings and by that they increase the oxygen intake during the night, resulting in less chance for snoring. They are non-invasive and do not require any special training, they are a portable solution, making them ideal for travel on-the-go use. They provide immediate relief from nasal congestion and improve sleep quality for both, snorer and their partner. They are a drug-free approach to reducing snoring, making them a safe option for most individuals. However they might seem to be as great solution, there is a small chance that they won't work, but this chance is very small.

Power of nasal breathing

“For breath is life, and if you breathe well you will live long on earth”

- Sanskrit Proverb

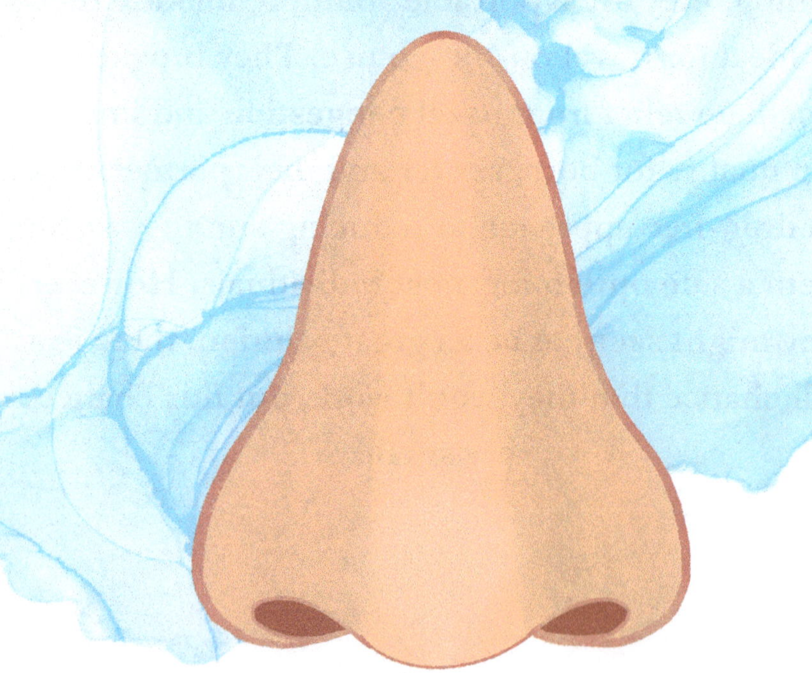

Nose breathing seems like a simple thing, but when you take the time to breathe through your nose, you're actually doing your body a lot of good. Nose breathing is a natural way to breathe that many people don't think about. It's the way we were designed to breathe and it has the key benefits for our health.

Our nose is designed to help you breathe safely, efficiently, and properly. Nose breathing imposes approximately 50% more resistance to the air stream, as compared to mouth breathing. This results in 10 to 20% more oxygen uptake. This is because when we breathe, the air travels through the small and large airways in the nose, which warms and humidifies the air before it enters the lungs. This means, that we get more oxygen with each breath.

Nose breathing can also help with weight loss. When we're stressed, we tend to breathe more quickly and shallowly, which can cause us to gain weight. if we practice nose breathing, it's going to help us to relax and control our stress levels, which might help us to lose weight in the long run.

Studies have shown that people who practice deep breathing, including nose breathing, have a lower risk of developing cancer. This is because deep breathing helps to improve the function of the immune system and circulates oxygen and blood to the body's tissues.

Nose breathing offers many health benefits that mouth breathing does not. For example, the nose filters heat and humidifies the air as it passes through the nasal cavity.

Breathing through your nose helps your body defend itself from bacteria. The little hairs in your nose, also known as cilia, are one of the biggest air filters in your body. As the air travels through your nose. It is then filtered through your sinuses, which are filled with a thick mucous membrane that traps any bacteria before the air continues to your lungs.

It cools or warms the air you breathe before it enters your lungs. Inferior turbinates build a heating and cooling system in your nose, they as well humidify and filter the air that we breathe.
Breathing through your nose enhances your lung and brain function, because you breathe more slowly, allowing your lungs to take more time to expand than when you breathe through your mouth.

Since your lungs more expand when you breathe through your nose, you are able to extract more oxygen from the air you breathe. This extra oxygen is distributed throughout your body and brain, allowing them to function better.

When we sleep, our body naturally alternates between breathing through the left and right nostrils, and through this process, regulates our body's functions, says rhinologist Dr. Belachew Tessema. Nose breathing improves sleep quality for a very simple reason. Sleep is one of the most important phases of your body during the day.

It's the only time when it has time to fully recharge and regenerate everything that was used during the day, all the organs, all the muscles, and all the cells are now free to fully rest while you are in a dreamland. Exactly at this very moment, the body needs the correct amount of oxygen that comes only by nose breathing. It's important at this moment to have the nose fully open and ready for all the possible oxygen it can breathe in.

Slower nose breathing activates the parasympathetic nervous system, reducing anxiety and signaling the body to calm down. Because it's the most natural way for our body to breathe, we put our state of mind into the best situation. The brain feels safe because this is a sign that you are at ease and there is no danger for you, all the chemicals in your body start positively flowing around, and regeneration and healing take place as well.

Nasal breathing is associated with more relaxed breathing, and lowering our blood pressure benefits our cardiovascular health. Losing this normal physiological function, shows up in different ways in different people, for some people that's high blood pressure, and for others, it's headaches, etc...

Nasal breathing is a powerful tool that can enhance athletes health and performance at nearly zero cost to coaches or athletes. Thanks to nasal breathing our body has up to 20% higher oxygen intake, which then can protect all of the muscles more from cramps or injury. That's one of the reasons why nasal breathing improves athletic performance and endurance. Slow and controlled nasal breathing is a communication of safety to the deepest parts of the nervous system, which is essential for progress and to increase the force we give out.

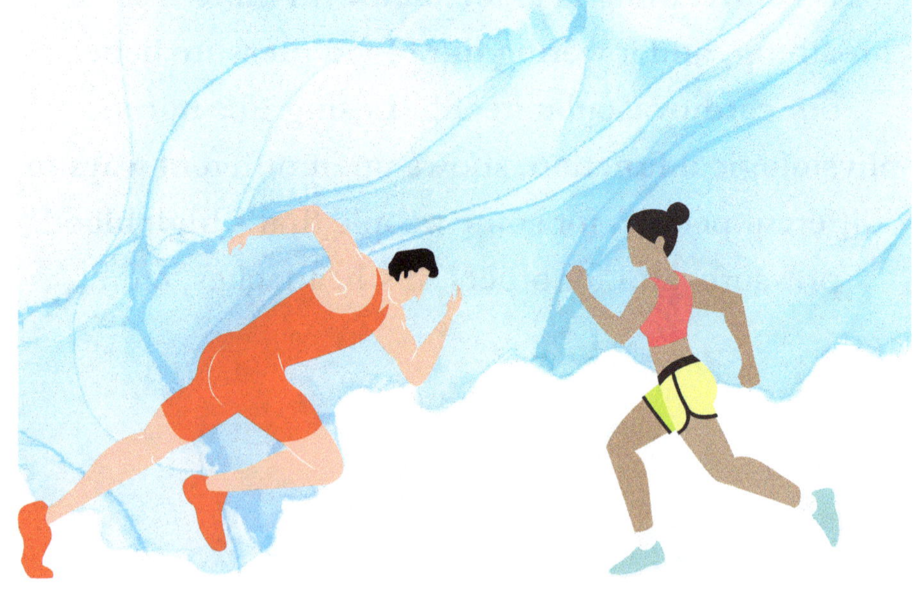

When we are stressed or anxious, our breathing tends
to be irregular and shallow. Deep breathing/
conscious breathing is a practice that enables more
airflow into our body and can help calm our nerves,
reducing anxiety, depression, and stress. It also helps
to improve our attention span and lower pain levels.
By taking shallow and short breaths from our chest,
we can induce a state of anxiety or panic.
That means that purposeful deep breathing can
physically calm our body down if we are feeling
stressed or anxious.

Our autonomic nervous system, which controls
involuntary actions like heart rate and digestion, is
split into two parts. One part, the sympathetic
nervous system, controls your fight or flight response.
The other part, the parasympathetic nervous system,
controls your rest and relaxation response.
It is not possible to turn the sympathetic nervous
system off completely, but shifting one's breathing to
a modulated, slow, relaxed pattern of not overly deep
inhales and exhales is a way to turn the volume down
on it.

One of the ways is that relaxed breathing patterns seem to calm the nervous system that controls the body's involuntary functions. Controlled breathing can cause physiological changes that include: lowered blood pressure and heart rate.

Deep breathing may be simple but it isn't necessarily easy, it can quit the nervous system in a short amount of time, though it probably won't provide instant relief from all anxiety. The more you practice, the better you'll get at it and the more you'll be able to use it in times of stress to help calm yourself down.

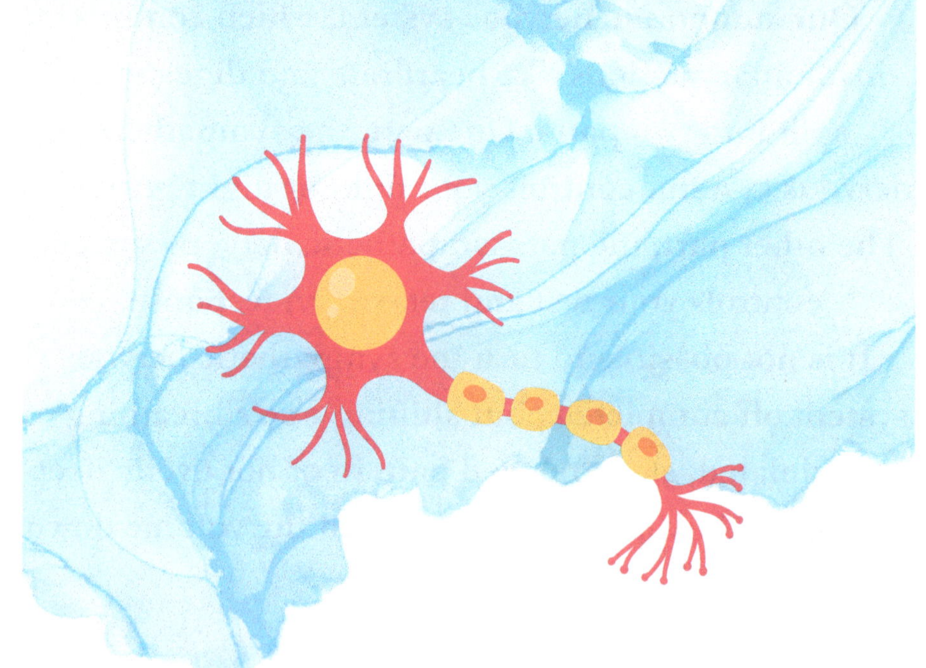

There are many ways to breathe deeply and various techniques have the power to ease up your mental troubles and let your mind rather flow than be destroyed by itself. Be kind to yourself as you practice deep breathing. Recognize that you might not notice results immediately, and that's completely okay. Give yourself credit for trying, and keep practicing, even just for a minute or two at a time, until your reach a point where you notice it's starting to help you manage your stress. Then keep at it. Deep breathing isn't like riding a bike, you must do it regularly for it to be helpful.

Watch yourself during the process, and observe and study your emotions and thinking patterns. Let the thoughts just be, don't judge them, don't give them any label, and let them flow in and out. At this moment you are in a state of gathering, gathering information about yourself and your body's responses. This is a very important process for your life and well-being.

Breathwork techniques

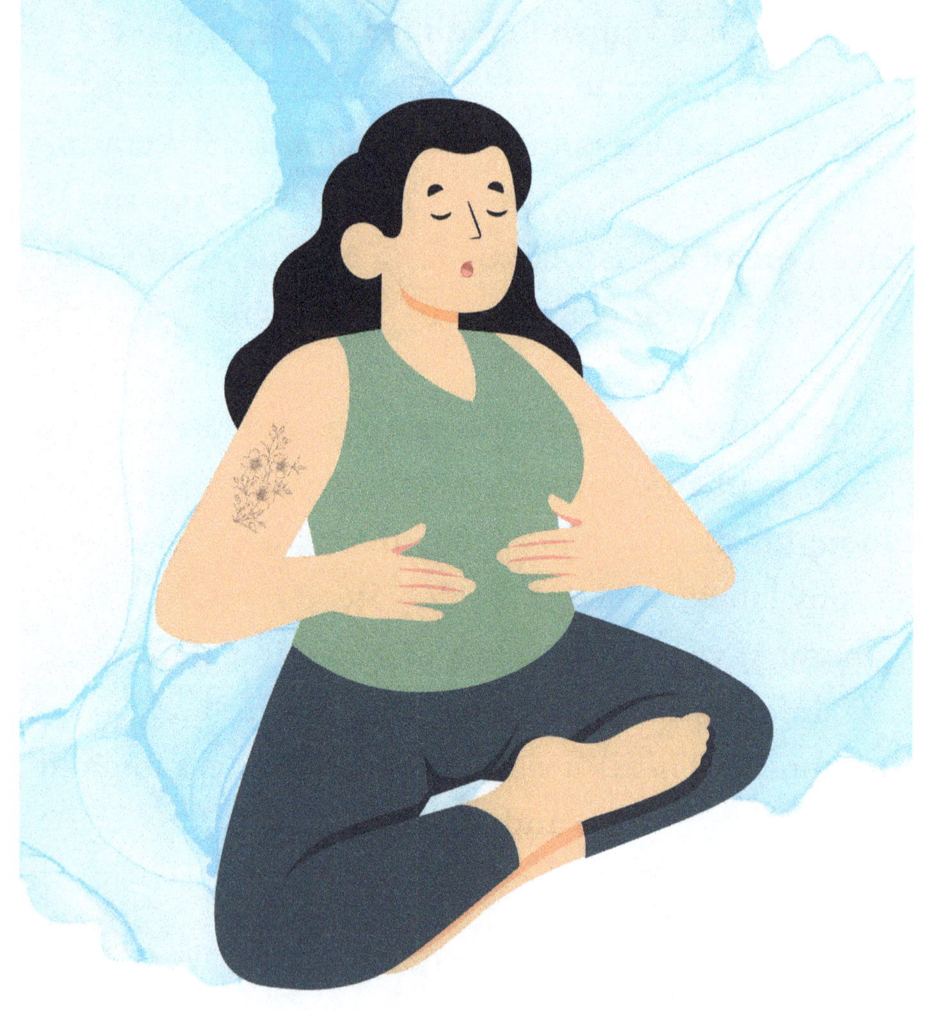

Box breathing

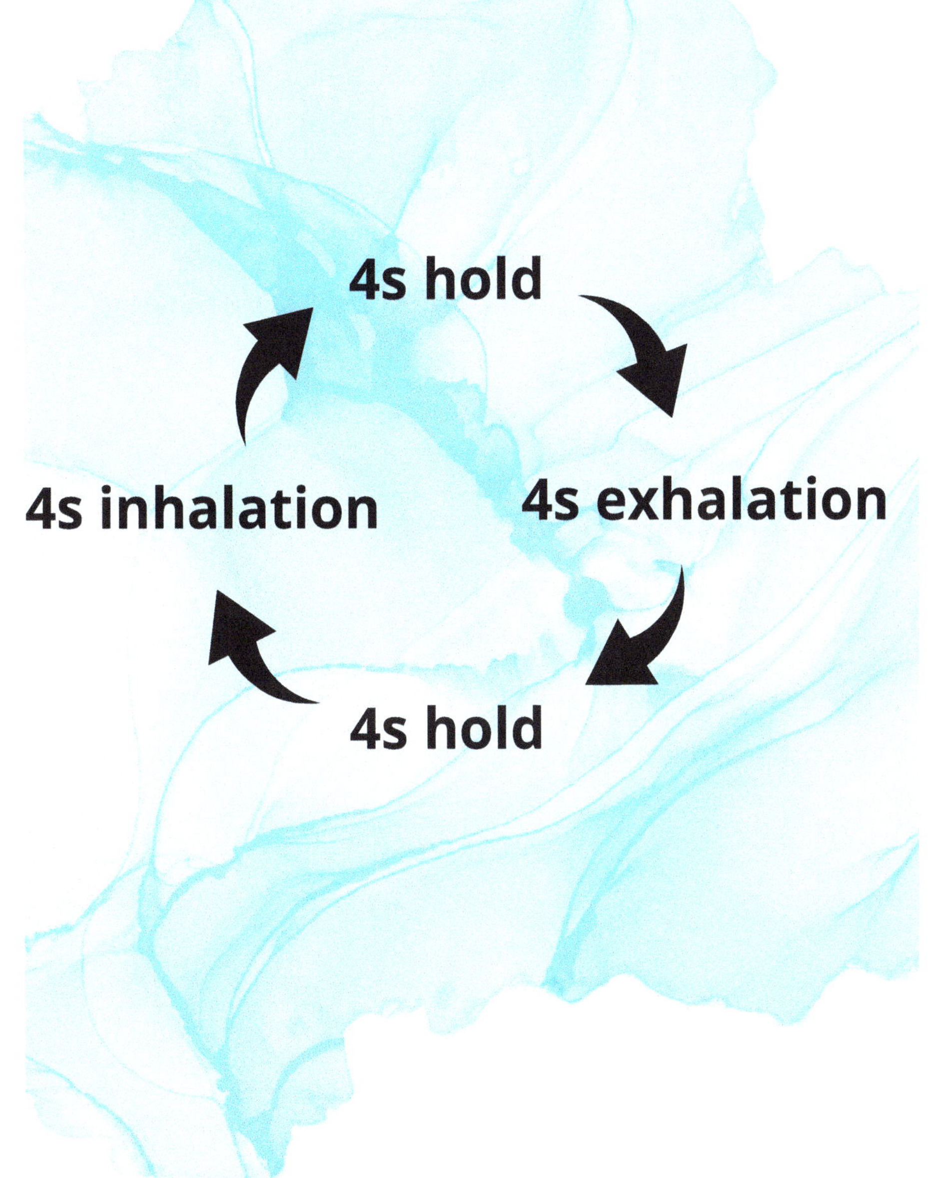

Also known as square breathing or 4-4-4-4 breathing, is a technique that helps to focus on taking slow, deep breaths. It's used by a wide variety of professionals and athletes for stress reduction and improved performance.

Box breathing was developed by Mark Divine, a former Navy SEAL commander, who has been using the technique since 1987.

It's regularly used by people in high-stress environments due to its ability to turn off a person's fight or flight mode. Using this exercise is seen as a great method of relaxation since it distracts your mind from the stresses around you as you focus specifically on your breathwork.

Benefits

- Allows you to feel calm and regulate your autonomic nervous system.
- Can help to regulate body temperature.
- Can help lower blood pressure.
- Reduces stress and improves mood, and can even assist in treating anxiety, panic disorder, PTSD, and depression.
- Can help treat insomnia when practiced before bed.
- Can help with pain management.

Here is how to do it:

1. To prepare for this exercise, sit up straight and attempt to push the oxygen out of your lungs by breathing slowly out of your mouth
2. Slowly breathe in through your nose for a count of 4. Focus on the air filling your lungs.
3. Hold your breath for another count of 4.
4. Breathe out through your mouth for a third count of 4. Pay attention to the sensation of the air leaving your body.
5. Hold your breath again for a final count of 4.
6. Continue to repeat these steps as much as desired.

Diaphragmatic breathing

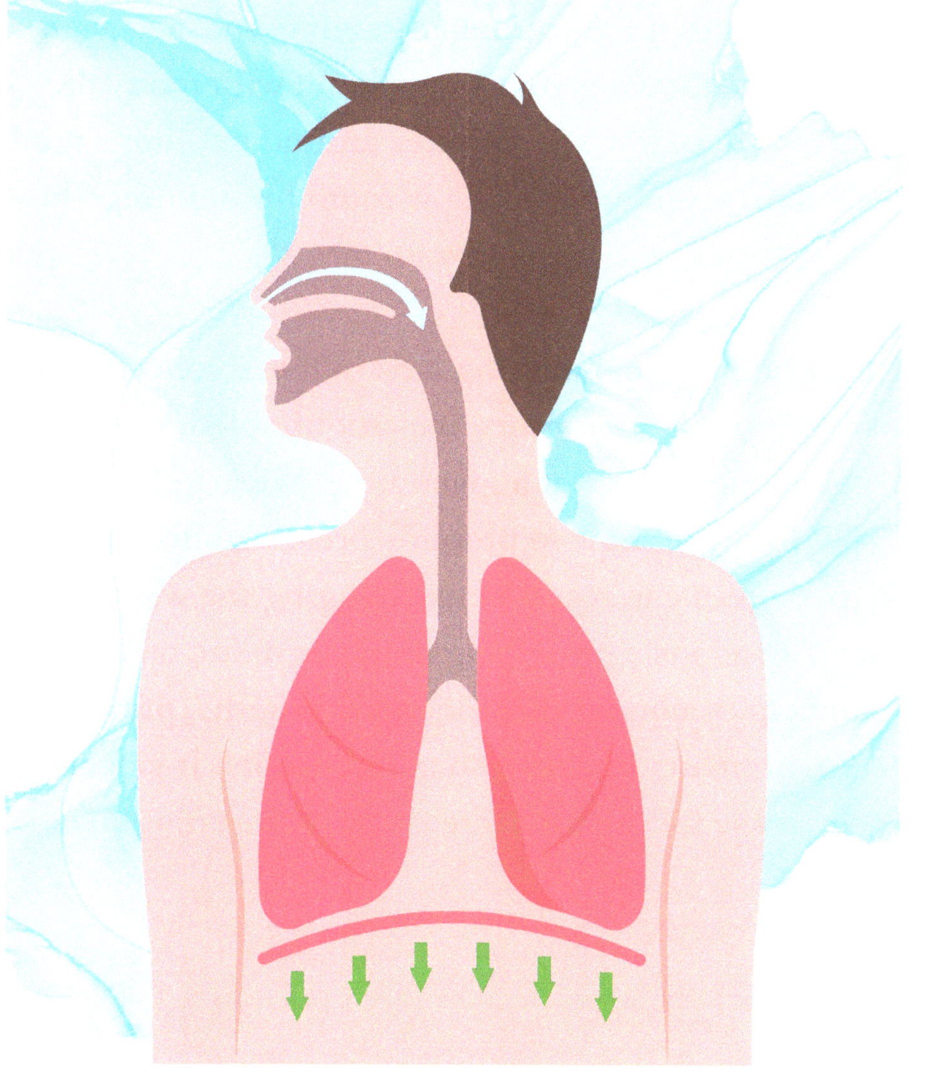

Also known as belly breathing or abdominal breathing, is breathwork that utilizes the stomach, abdomen, and diaphragm. It works by using your muscles to force your diaphragm to move as you breathe, allowing your lungs to fill with more air. When we breathe, the muscles around our lungs tend to contract in order to allow room for our lungs to expand with air.

Diaphragmatic breathing aids in these contractions in order to help improve the amount of air that can enter your lungs at a given time. We are all born knowing how to properly breathe, but life experiences can result in us changing the way we do so. Consciously practicing diaphragmatic breathing can help us correct these learned patterns, providing us with many improved health benefits. It can also increase focus and decrease negative emotions.

Benefits:

- helps to correct your breathing patterns
- Improves your ability to tolerate intense exercise
- Lowers chances of injuring or wearing out your muscles
- Creates a sense of relaxation and lowers stress levels
- Improves concentration levels
- Strengthens your diaphragm and improves core muscle stability.
- Reduces oxygen demand by lowering heart rate and blood pressure
- Assists with anxiety, depression, PTSD, COPD, IBS, sleeplessness, and asthma.

Here is how to do it:

- Sit in a comfortable position or lie down on a flat surface. You can sit on a pillow or place them under your head and knees to keep you comfortable.
- Relax your shoulders.
- Place one hand on your upper chest.
- Place the other hand on your stomach between the rib cage and diaphragm.
- Slowly breathe in through your nose. Focus on drawing the air down towards your stomach as you push it against your hand. Try to keep your chest still.
- Tighten your abdominal muscles and let your stomach fall while pressing downward as you breathe out through your lips. Continue to try to keep your chest still.
- Continue to inhale and exhale as desired.

Pursed lip breathing

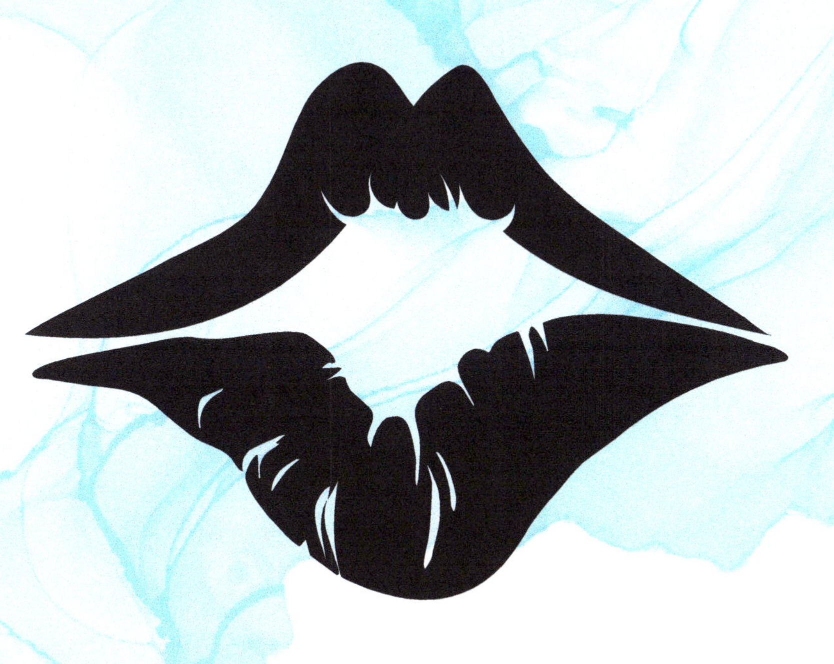

Involves slowly breathing in and out through pursed lips. This is a technique used to give more control over your breath and ultimately make your breath more impactful. Pursed lip breathing has been shown to strengthen your lungs with regular practice. This technique focuses on slowing your breath and emptying stale air from your lungs, which is beneficial for those struggling with chronic lung disease and other conditions.

A 2018 study, exploring the effects of pursed lip breathing showed improvements among patients with **COPD**. It's also an effective aid when accomplishing difficult physical tasks, such as climbing the stairs. It should be noted that this technique works best when you're already relaxed.

Benefits:

- Relieves shortness of breath.
- Reduces the work required to breathe.
- Removes carbon trapped in your lungs and brings in more fresh air
- Assists with conditions that make it difficult to breathe, including asthma, pulmonary fibrosis, and **COPD**.

4-7-8 breathing technique

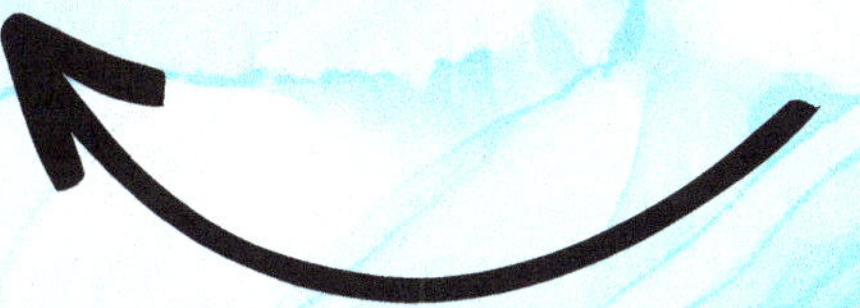

This technique is another technique that promotes relaxation. As a result, it has been successful in regulating the flight or fight response and helping to combat stress and anxiety. By forcing you to focus on your breaths rather than your worries, it helps to achieve a state of calm and more easily fall asleep.

Benefits:

- Helps control mood and improves stress and anxiety levels.
- Assists in falling asleep and decreases fatigue.
- Reduces cravings.
- Reduces asthma symptoms...
- Reduces hypertension.
- Improves migraine symptoms.

Here is how to do it:

1. As you part your lips, breathe out through your mouth while making a whooshing sound.
2. Close your mouth and inhale through your nose to the count of 4.
3. Hold your breath for a count of 7.
4. Make another whooshing sound as you breathe out your mouth for a count of 8.
5. Repeat these steps as much as desired.

Alternate nostril breathing

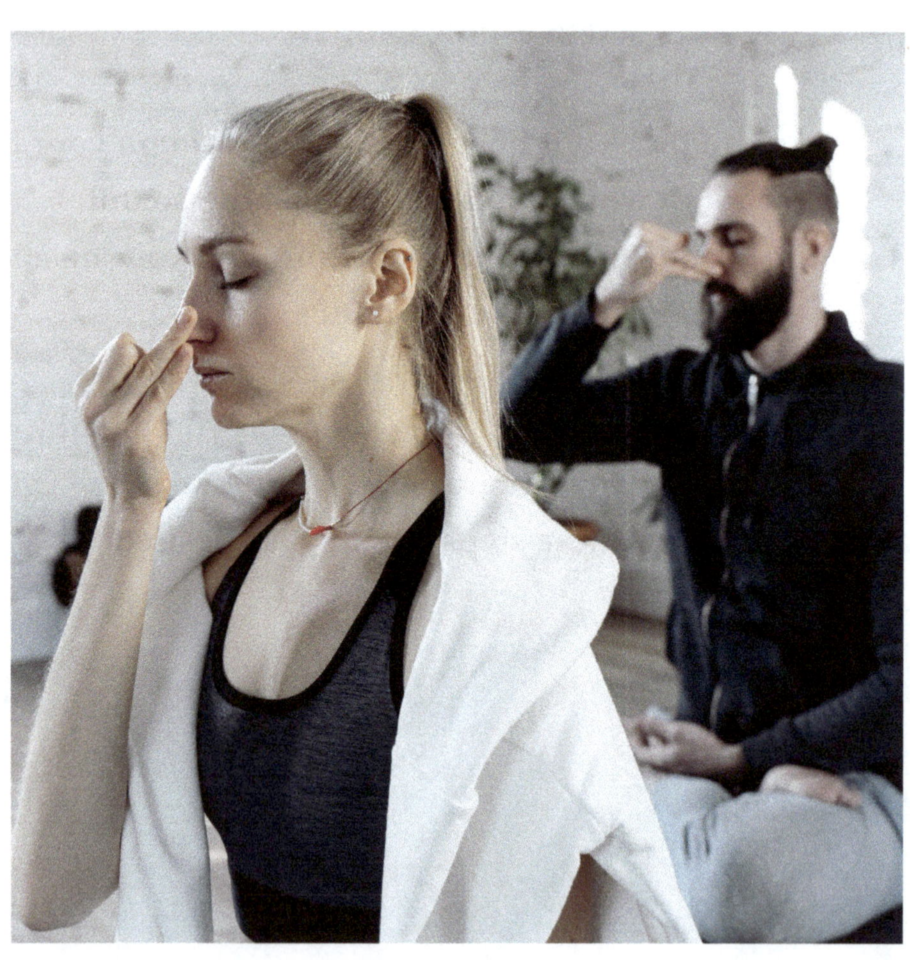

Is an exercise that allows you to practice breath control. It is often done during yoga or meditation, and it can also be practiced as part of pranayama breathwork. Alternate nostril breathing works under the knowledge that the left nostril increases activity in the right side of your brain while breathing through the right nostril increases activity in the left. While the right side of our brain is responsible for emotions and creativity, the left side is responsible for logic and language. By breathing through both sides equally, you help to stimulate both parts of your brain. Might be also effective for lowering stress levels.

Benefits:

- Allows for relaxation.
- Reduces stress and anxiety.
- Improves cardiovascular health, including heart rate.
- Improves lung function and respiratory endurance.
- Enhances overall physical and mental health.

Here is how to do it:

1. Sit down with your legs crossed.
2. Place your left hand on your left knee and lift your right hand up to your nose.
3. Breathe out, then close your right nostril with your right thumb.
4. Breathe in through your left nostril, then use your fingers to close it.
5. Release your thumb from your right nostril and breathe out through this side.
6. Breathe in through your right nostril, then close it again with your thumb.
7. Release your fingers from your left nostril and breathe out through this side. You've now completed a full cycle.
8. Repeat as much as desired, being sure to end on a completed cycle.

The Breath of Now

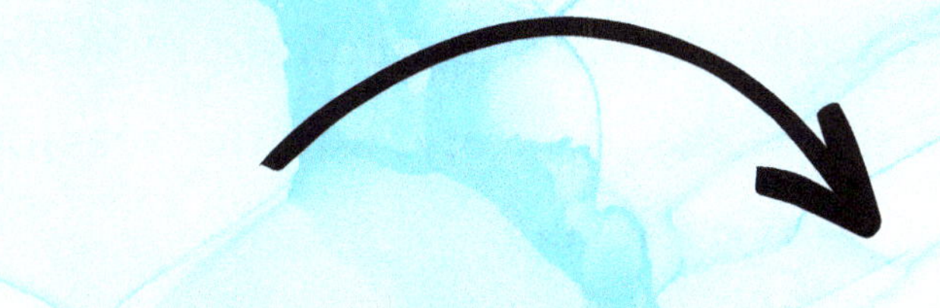

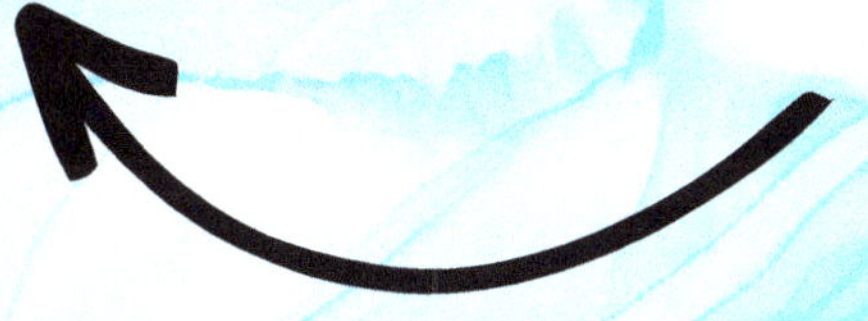

Also known as the moment. It's conscious nose breathing combined with tongue press awareness. This is a simple and easy exercise that can be done by anyone, anywhere, and almost under any circumstances. This breathing technique instantly decreases the stress, anxiety, and depression levels.

Allowing your nervous system to reset and clear your mind from the feeling of being overwhelmed by all of the thoughts. An important part of this practice is to fully concentrate on the tongue pressing to the roof of your mouth and counting up to 5 seconds while you do that. Feel fully the pressure you feel, become the pressure itself.

Benefits:

- Resets your nervous system
- Calms your mind
- Allows you to access more creative thinking
- Reduces stress, anxiety and depression

Here is how it works:

- Sit, lay, or stand in a comfortable and safe position
- Place your tongue on the roof of your mouth, and touch with the tip of the tongue the back of the teeth
- Press the tongue against the roof as you inhale, counting up to 5 seconds
- Quickly and deeply exhale
- Continue for 1 minute
- Take a 30-second break and let your tongue muscles and jaw rest.
- Repeat the cycle at least 3 times

Breath focus technique

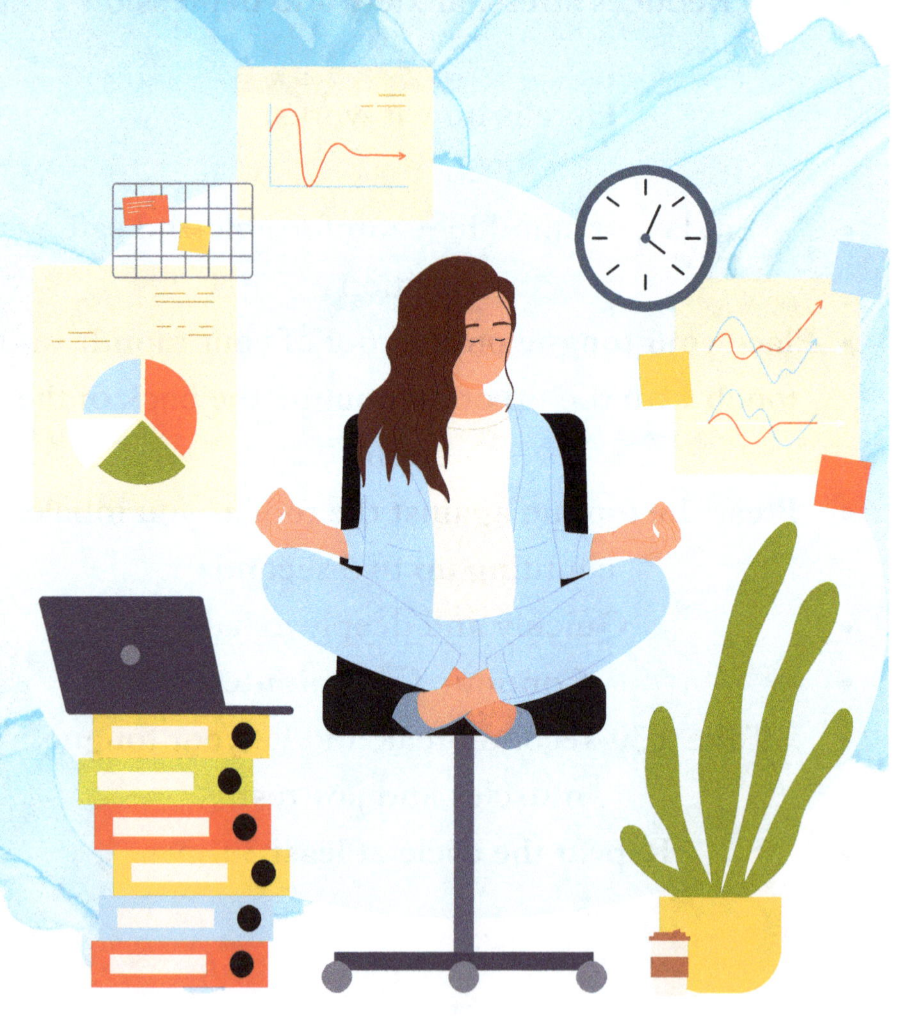

Also known as mindful breathing, is a technique that has practitioners focus on imagery, words, or phrases. These images or words will often be ones that contribute to feelings of happiness, relaxation, or neutrality.

The breath focus technique is common to yoga, meditation, and various therapies for its ability to help with stress reduction. it's believed that focusing on your breath can lead to positive physical and mental changes.

A study by the Journal of Neurophysiology, recently showed that the regions of our brain linked to emotions, attention, and body awareness actually light up when we engage in focused breathing. Additional studies showed that it can be used for stress reduction based on the areas of the brain that light up during rapid breathing and focused breathing

Benefits:

- Reduces stress and anxiety
- Increase alertness and improves concentration
- Boosts your immune system
- Increases vitality

Here is how to do it:

- Sit or lie down in a comfortable position.
- Pay attention to the way you're breathing. Try not to change the way you breathe prior to this technique.
- Switch between normal breathing and deep breathing a few times, paying attention to how they differ from each other and how your abdomen moves.
- Take a few shallow breaths, noticing how they differ from your deep breaths.
- Continue to deep breathe for a few more minutes.
- Place a hand below your belly button as you relax your stomach. Pay attention to how it rises and falls as you continue to breathe.

- Every time you breathe out, let out a loud sigh.
- As you continue to breathe deeply, begin to focus on a relaxing image, word, or phrase of your choice.
- Imagine the air you breathe in is a wave bringing peace and calm into your body. You can mentally say "inhaling peace and calmness" as you do this.
- As you breathe out, picture any negativity you're feeling being washed away. You can mentally say "exhaling tension and anxiety" as you do this.
- You have now completed a breath of focus session.

Equal breathing

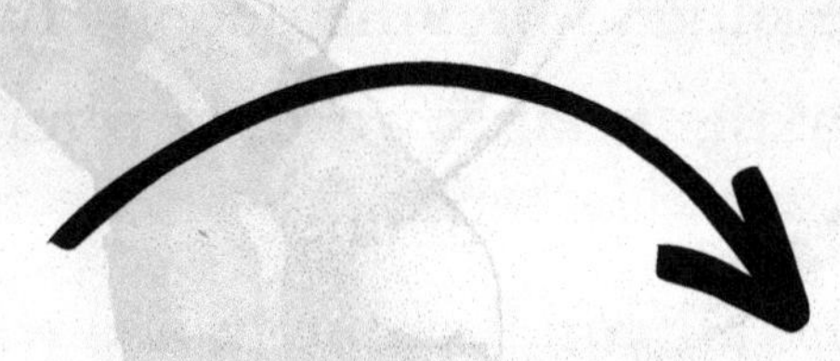

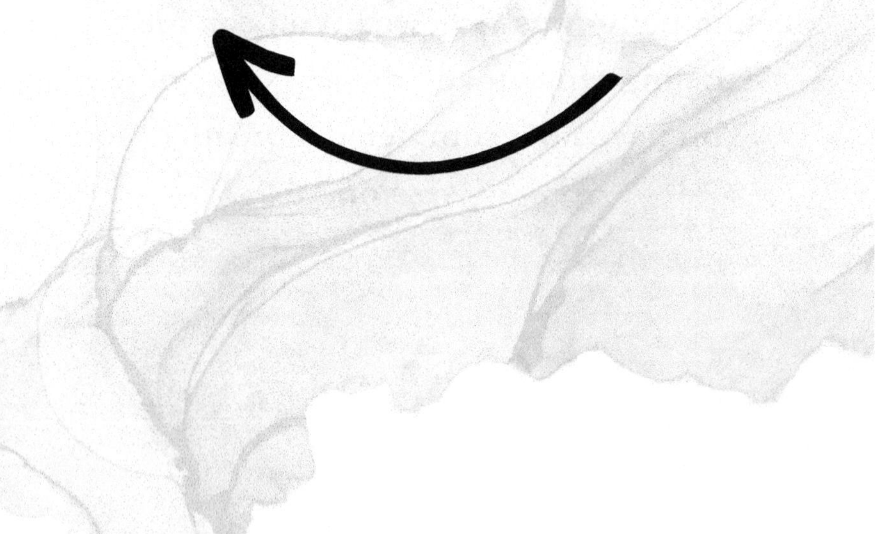

Also known as circular breathing or Sama Vritti, is an exercise that focuses on making your inhales and exhales the same length. This is done to make your breath smooth and steady and to help you achieve a sense of balance and equanimity. Equal breathing engages your parasympathetic nervous system, which helps you to achieve relaxation.

It works well for those looking to ease their stress and anxiety quickly, which was documented in a 2017 study. It's also recommended as an exercise prior to going to bed since it works similarly to counting sheep. This is because it helps you to focus on measuring your breath instead of any of the racing thoughts in your head.

Benefits:

- Calms your nerves
- Improves your focus and concentration
- Helps to quiet the mind
- Allows you to access your full breathing capacity

Here is how it works:

1. Sit down in a comfortable position.
2. Breathe in and out through your nose.
3. Count your inhales and exhales to make sure that they are the same length. If this is uneasy, select a word or phrase to mentally say with every inhale and exhale.
4. You can also take a short pause between each inhale and exhale if this is helpful.
5. Continue this exercise for as long as desired.

Resonant or coherent breathing

5 breaths

Also known as coherent breathing, is when one breathes at a rate of 5 breaths per minute. This is one of the simple exercises that can be done anywhere at any time. A study determined that resonant breathing improves heart rate and mood. Since resonant breathing is designed to help you breathe at 5 breaths per minute, this allows you to maximize your heart rate variability. Since your heart rate is linked to your nervous system, you can easily improve your HRV with breathwork and also calm your nerves. This helps relieve stress.

Benefits:

- **Regulates the autonomic nervous system.**
- **Reduces stress and anxiety and can relieve depression symptoms.**
- **Helps control blood pressure.**
- **Relieves symptoms related to asthma, COPD, fibromyalgia, and IBS.**
- **Can help treat insomnia.**

Here is how to do it:

1. Get into a comfortable position of your choice.
2. **Breathe in for a count of 5.**
3. **Breathe out for a count of 5.**
4. **Continue these steps as desired.**

Supplemental oxygen A.K.A. Oxygen therapy

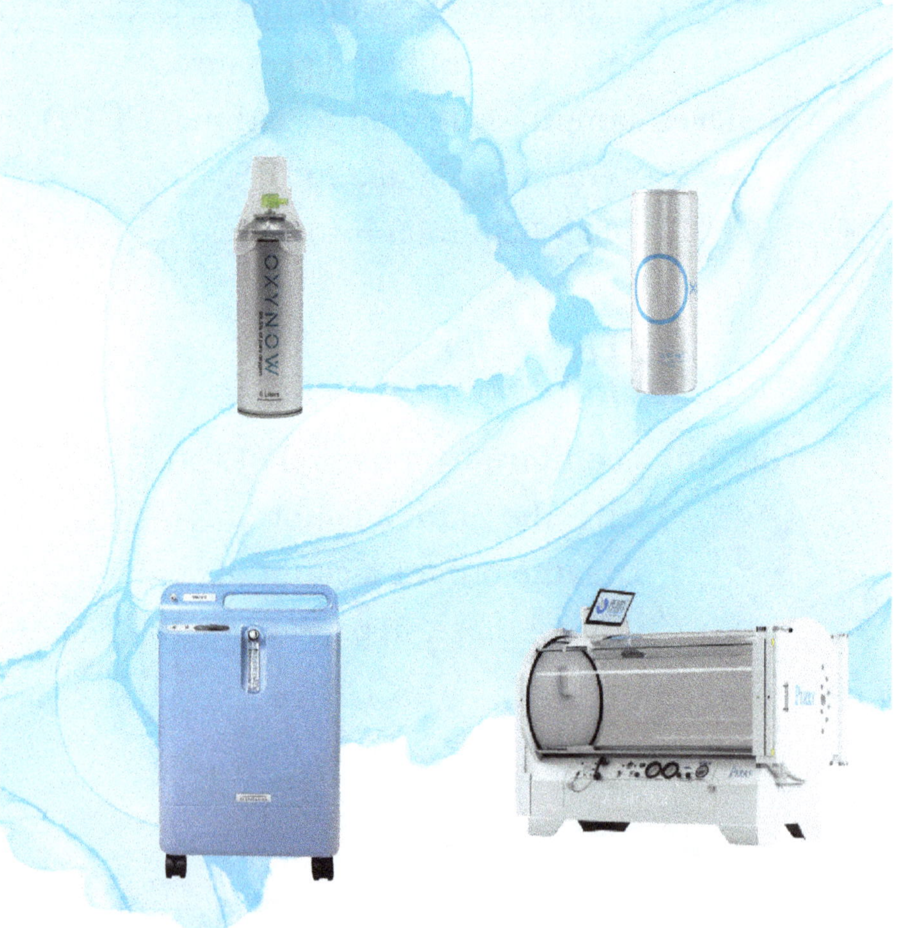

What is it, how it works, why it might be beneficial for you to use it?

Learning all you can about oxygen therapy can help you feel more comfortable and confident about its usage.

Our lungs absorb oxygen from the air. When we inhale, oxygen begins to be absorbed into our body already in the nose thanks to the mucous membrane. It then continues to our lungs, where it is fully absorbed into our body using the alveoli. In the alveoli of the lungs, it binds to hemoglobin, which is in red blood platelets. They will deliver a new dose of energy to muscles, organs, and all parts of our body.

Oxygen therapy is often used in hospitals for faster recovery after various operations or for patients with breathing difficulties. For example, it has a positive effect on patients after general anesthesia. The simplest form of oxygen therapy is oxygen concentrators, which suck in ambient air. The oxygen concentrator then enriches this air with pure oxygen and it is then transported through our nasal airways to the whole body through an oxygen cannula or a breathing mask.

Oxygen therapy is a treatment that provides you with supplemental, or extra oxygen. It can help you feel better and stay active. Although oxygen therapy may be common in the hospital, it can also be used at home. There are several devices used to deliver oxygen at home. Supplemental oxygen does not cure lung disease, but it is an important therapy that improves symptoms and organ functions.

Oxygen therapy can help you by decreasing shortness of breath or breathlessness
Oxygen therapy won't completely take away your shortness of breath, but it can help many lung disease patients feel less breathless during everyday activities.

Not everyone who has shortness of breath is a candidate for oxygen, so be sure to talk to your doctor about whether it is right for you.

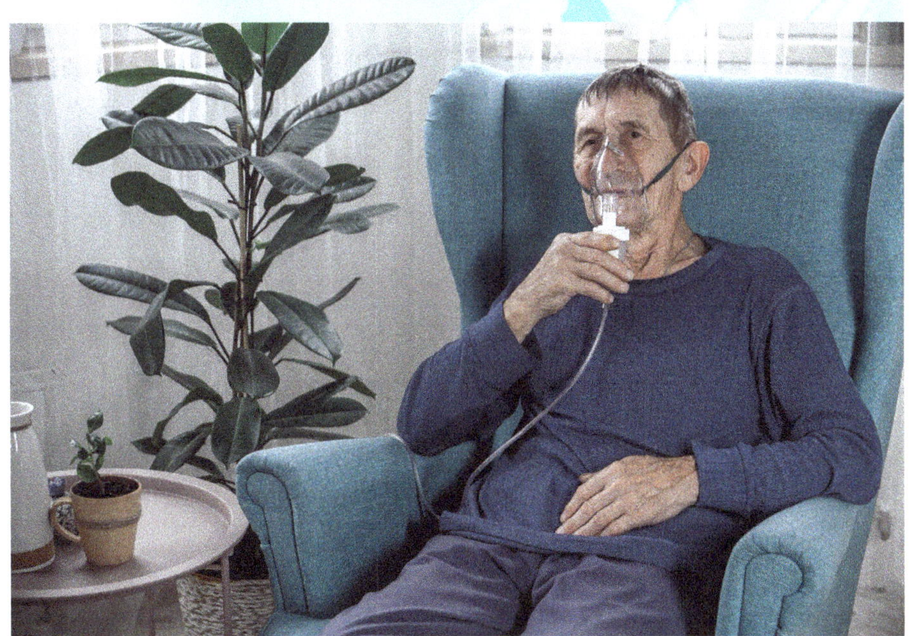

Less fatigue

The low percentage of oxygen inside your body might make you feel exhausted and tired. There for simple tasks such as household chores, walking stairs, and interacting with friends can be a struggle. Oxygen therapy circulates more oxygen into your bloodstream, which is improving your energy levels.

Sleep better

People with lung disease often have a hard time sleeping or don't get very restful sleep. There are many reasons for this, but one is that people with lung disease lose oxygen in their blood overnight, especially during REM sleep. Using oxygen therapy at night allows your body to get more oxygen into the bloodstream so that you may get a better night's sleep. Using oxygen therapy over the night is something to be consulted with your doctor.

More energy

Oxygen therapy may help you become more active and get you back to doing the activities you enjoy. When your body has enough oxygen, you will have more energy to be more active. Staying active is a key part of staying healthy as possible.

Oxygen therapy might be used as a medical or recreational tool. They are different in style and time of usage.
Oxygen therapy is used recreationally by athletes, everyday people, people working in stressful environments, managers, pregnant women, seniors, students, and children.

Oxygen therapy during sports

The use of oxygen therapy in sports circles is nothing new. It has been used for decades for its beneficial effects and positive effects on the body. With each training session, we discover the true magic and benefits of oxygen therapy.

Up to 90% of our energy comes from oxygen, which makes this element the most important of all elements known to us. The Polish alchemist and doctor Michal Sendivoj called oxygen the "Food of Life".

What are the positive effects of oxygen therapy in the case of recreational use?

- Energy Boost
- Higher dynamics
- Accelerated cell regeneration
- Decreasing levels of stress, anxiety, and depression
- Higher quality fetal nutrition during pregnancy
- Increasing concentration
- It has a positive effect against migraines or spasms
- Helps with shortness of breath and difficulty breathing in the elderly

For a beginner user of recreational oxygen therapy using oxygen concentrators, we recommend starting with 15-30 minutes a day, 3 times a week. Proper hydration is important, it helps the overall body functioning.

During oxygen therapy, watch how your body reacts and gradually increase the intensity according to the feeling. It is ideal to always have a 1-day break between therapy. The time of use should not exceed more than 1 hour on a single day.

The use of oxygen therapy cannot in any case exceed the inhalation period of more than 24 hours. Unless it is not prescribed by your specialist or doctor for your specific problem. If you are unsure about using oxygen therapy, always consult your medical professional.

Air pollution

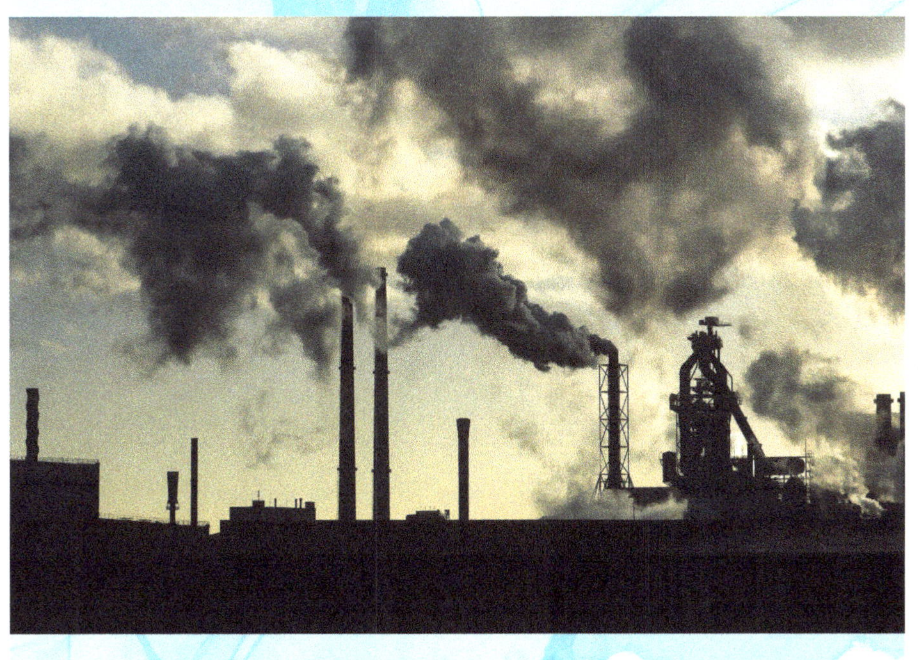

Air pollution is the contamination of the indoor or outdoor environment by any chemical, physical or biological agent that modifies the natural characteristic of the atmosphere.

Household combustion devices, motor vehicles, industrial facilities, and forest fires are common sources of air pollution. Pollutants of major public health concern include particulate matter, carbon monoxide, ozone, nitrogen dioxide, and sulfur dioxide. Outdoor and indoor air pollution cause respiratory and other diseases and are important sources of morbidity and mortality.

WHO data show that almost all of the global population (99%) breathe air that exceeds WHO guideline limits and contents high levels of pollutants, with low and middle-income countries suffering from the highest exposures.

Air quality

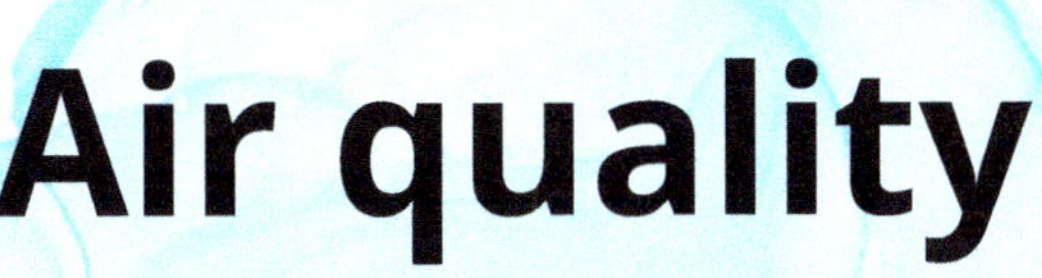

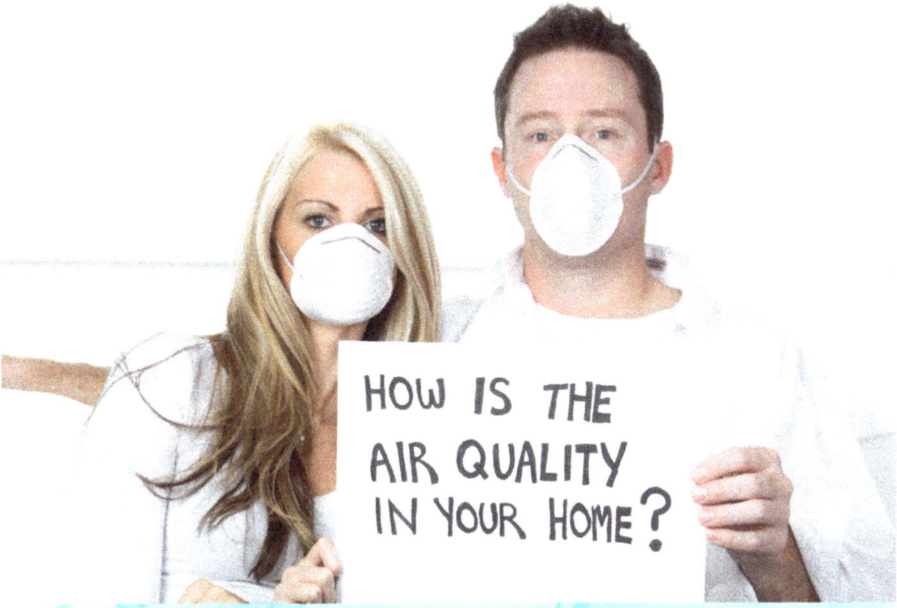

The first question you might ask is, why does air quality change?

Because air is always moving and that's why it can change from day to day or even from hour to hour. For a specific location, the air quality is a direct result of both, how air moves through the area and how people are influencing it.

How do humans influence the air?

Mountain ranges, coastlines, or land that was modified by people can cause air pollutants to concentrate in, or disperse from an area. The amounts of pollutants entering the air have a way larger impact on air quality. There might be also other pollutants in the form of natural forces such as volcanic activity or dust storms, but most of the pollutants come from human activity. Vehicles, coal-burning power plants, or toxic gases from industry. These are just a few examples of human-made air pollutants, the list goes on and on.

A huge role here plays the wind, which moves the air pollution around. A coastal area with an inland mountain range may have more air pollution during the day when sea breezes push pollutants over the land and lower air pollution in the evening because the direction of the breeze reserves and pushes air pollution out over the ocean.

Another thing that affects air quality is temperature. In urban areas, air quality is often worse in the winter months. When the air temperature is cooler, exhaust pollutants can be trapped close to the surface beneath a layer of dense, cold air.

Air pollution negatively impacts the land and ocean as well as the air we breathe every day. That's why good air quality is critical for maintaining healthy human, animal, and plant life on Earth. With the fact that 80% of the world's energy budget comes from burning fossil fuels, air quality remains the top concern for our present and future quality of life.

Good quality air means the air is free of harmful substances. Air quality is rated using air quality categories, which rate the amount of pollution in the air based on airborne concentrations of major pollutants, the higher the AQC the poorer the air quality

An air pollutant is any substance in the air that can harm people or the environment. Air pollution is a health concern in Australia and around the World. It can be particularly critical to the health of children, older people, pregnant women, and people with pre-existing health conditions. It affects the natural and built environment and the liveability of our communities.

Pollutants arise from natural processes like bushfires and from human activities, such as industrial and transport processes. The common primary air pollutant is particulate matter, ozone, nitrogen dioxide, carbon monoxide, and sulfur dioxide.

Particulate matter is extremely small solid particles and liquid droplets suspended in the air. It can be made up of a variety of components including nitrates, sulfates, organic chemicals, metals, soil or dust particles, and allergens. Particulate pollution mainly comes from motor vehicles, wood-burning heaters, and industry, these are the most common that we meet in everyday life. Also during bushfires or dust storms it can reach extremely high concentrations.

Potential health effects from exposure to particulate matter

Numerous studies have shown associations between exposure to particles and increased hospital admissions as well as death from heart or lung diseases. Currently, there is no evidence of a threshold below which exposure to particulate matter does not cause any health effects. It can occur after both short and long-term exposure to particulate matter.

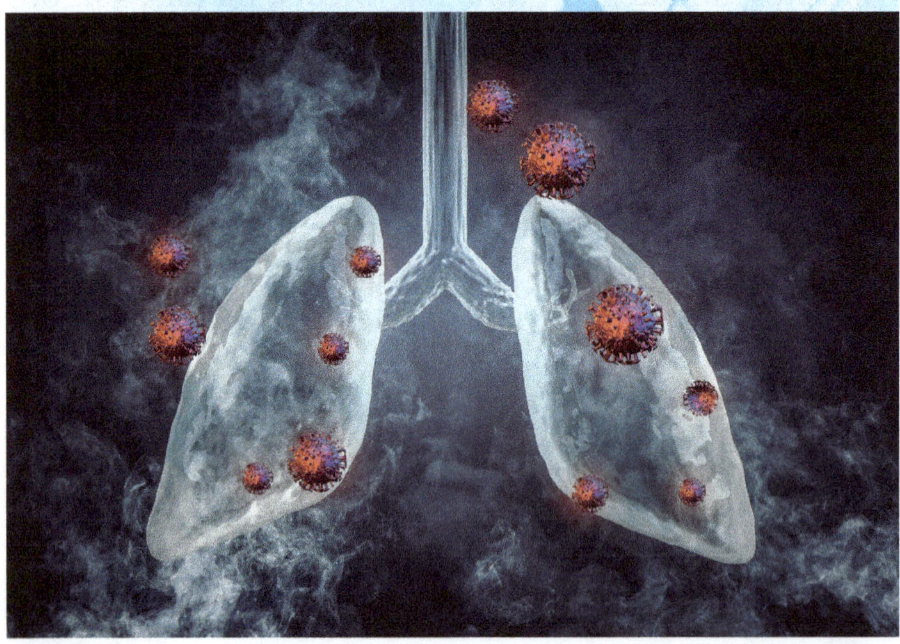

Short-term exposure can lead to:

Irritated eyes, nose, and throat
Worsening asthma and lung diseases such as chronic
bronchitis, heart attacks, and arrhythmias in people
with heart disease
Increases in hospital admissions and premature
death due to diseases of the respiratory and
cardiovascular systems

Long-term exposure can lead to:

Reduced lung function
Development of cardiovascular and respiratory
diseases
Increase rate of disease progression
Reduction in life expectancy

On the other hand, addressing air pollution requires a multifaceted approach involving government policies, technological advancement, and individual actions. Some potential solutions for air pollution include:

- Transitioning to clean energy: Promoting the use of renewable energy sources like solar, wind, and hydroelectric power can reduce the emissions from fossil fuel-based energy production, which is a major contributor to air pollution.
- Improving transportation: Encouraging the use of public transportation, electric vehicles and promoting active transportation options like walking and cycling can help reduce emissions from the transportation sector.
- Enhancing industrial processes: Implementing cleaner production methods and technologies in industries can significantly reduce emissions of harmful pollutants.

- Strengthening environmental regulations. enforcing and tightening emission standards for industries and vehicles can lead to cleaner air and improved public health.
- Forest conservation and afforestation: Protecting existing forests and planting more trees can help absorb and sequester carbon dioxide and other pollutants from the air.
- Waste management: Proper waste disposal and recycling practices can help reduce the release of harmful pollutants from landfills and waste incineration.
- Promoting green building design: Encouraging the construction of energy-efficient and sustainable buildings can reduce energy consumption and associated emissions.

- **Public awareness and education:** Increasing awareness about air pollution and its health impacts can foster a sense of responsibility among individuals, encouraging them to adopt cleaner practices.
- **International cooperation:** Collaborating on a global scale to address transboundary air pollution can help tackle regional air quality issues more effectively.
- **Research and innovation:** Investing in research and development of advanced technologies for cleaner energy production and pollution control can lead to long-term solutions.

Breath and oxygen are the most important
things that exist in our life.

Without breath and oxygen, there wouldn't
be any life. That's why it's important to be
mindful of breathing and take care of the
only thing we can breathe.

We cannot afford to lose THE OXYGEN.

Because without that we won't survive
longer, than 2 or 3 minutes. Think about that
for a second. In the time you read this text,
you already breathed 5 times.

#everybreathmatters

**This e-book was created and published by Oxynow s.r.o.
To spread awareness about the most important things on this planet.**

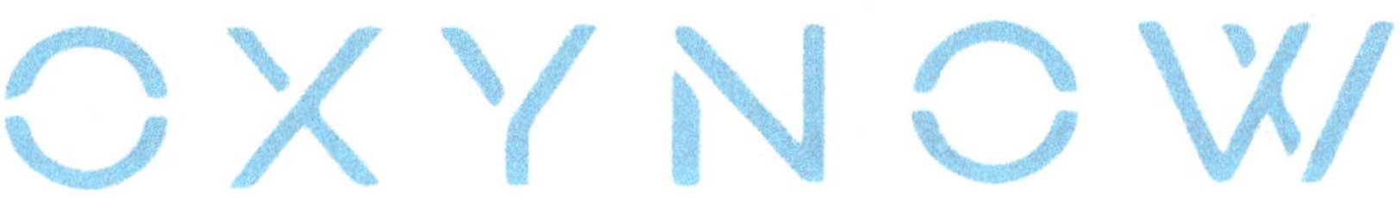

www.oxynowoxygen.com

Sources

https://www.brisbanebulkbillingdoctor.com.au/

https://www.oralhealthgroup.com/

https://www.ncbi.nlm.nih.gov/

https://www.healthline.com/

https://www.sciencedirect.com/

https://houstonadvancedsinus.com/

https://www.uhhospitals.org/

https://simplifaster.com/

The health benefits of nose breathing

https://www.medicalnewstoday.com/

https://www.othership.us/

https://rightasrain.uwmedicine.org/

https://www.mayoclinic.org/

https://www.sleepfoundation.org/

OXYGEN IS THE ONLY THING THAT PROVIDES US WITH LIFE. WITHOUT IT ALL LIFE WE KNOW IS LOST.

www.ingramcontent.com/pod-product-compliance
Lightning Source LLC
Chambersburg PA
CBHW071608270726
48661CB00019B/1645